MW01116249

A CUB COME TRUE

A Same Sex Family Building Story

By Drs. Pietro Bortoletto & Eduardo Hariton

This book is dedicated to our families and the ones we hope to help create for all of our patients. **99**

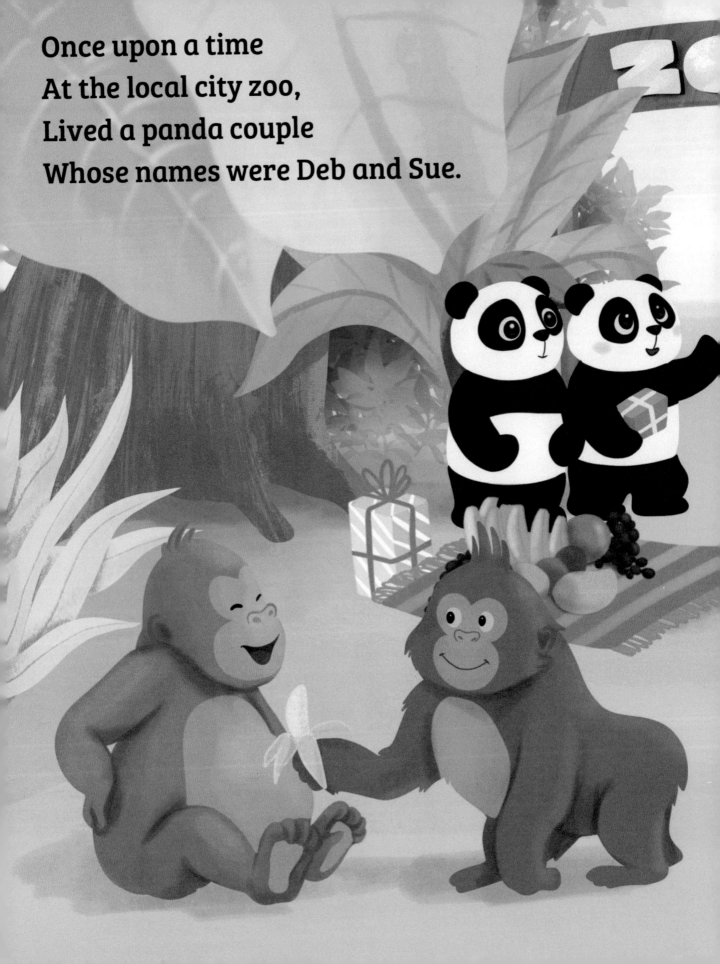

Once upon a time
At the local city zoo,
Lived a panda couple
Whose names were Deb and Sue.

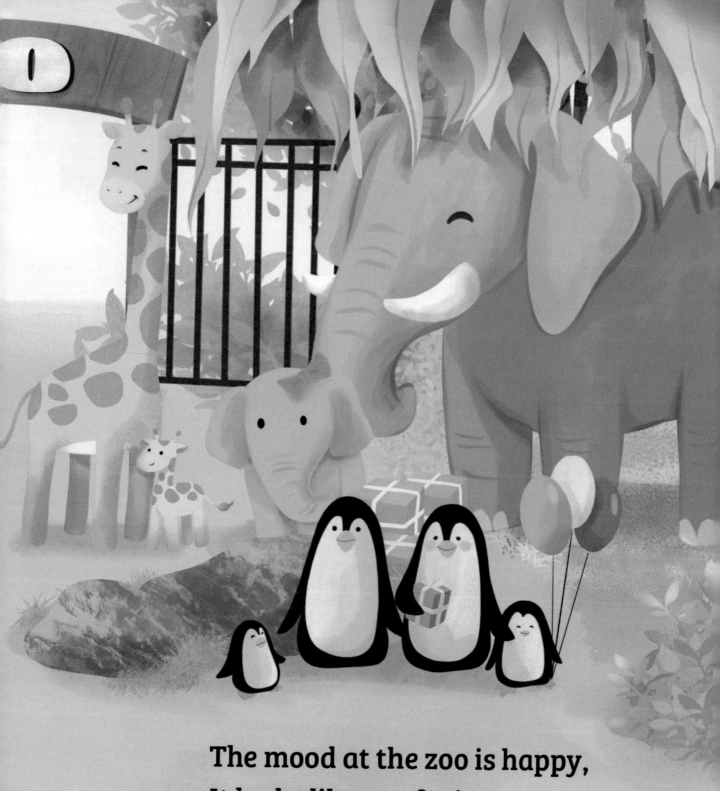

The mood at the zoo is happy,
It looks like a safari.
Today is the elephant couple's
Baby shower party!

Deb and Sue are smiling
But their hearts are sad inside.
They want to start a family
But the months keep passing by.

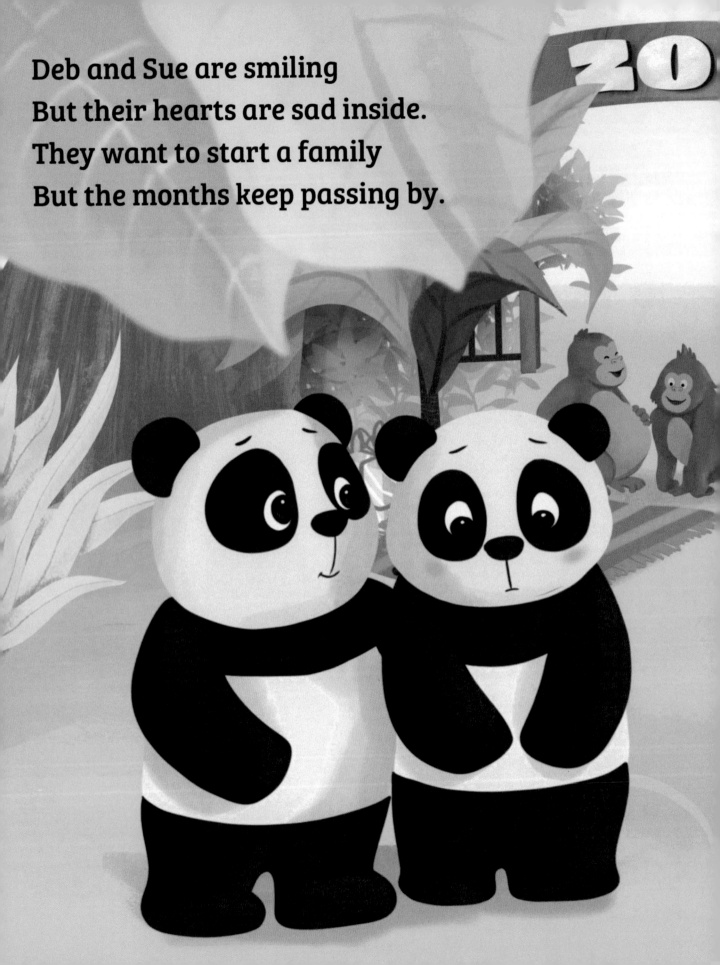

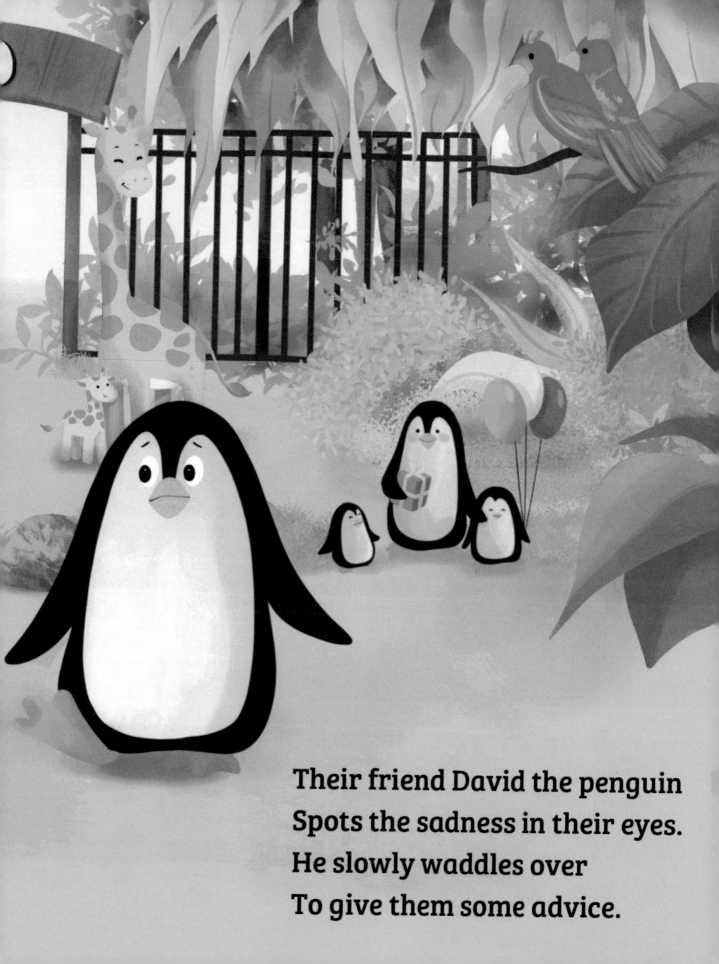

Their friend David the penguin
Spots the sadness in their eyes.
He slowly waddles over
To give them some advice.

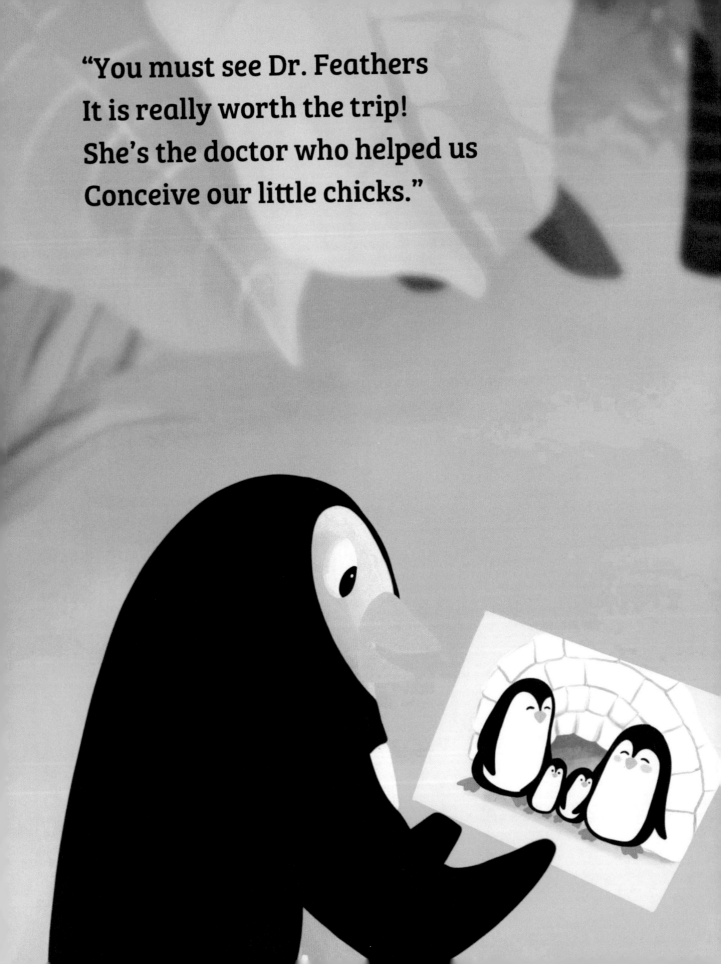

"You must see Dr. Feathers
It is really worth the trip!
She's the doctor who helped us
Conceive our little chicks."

Deb and Sue's eyes brighten
And their hopes grow more and more.
Could Dr. Feathers give them
The cub that they long for?

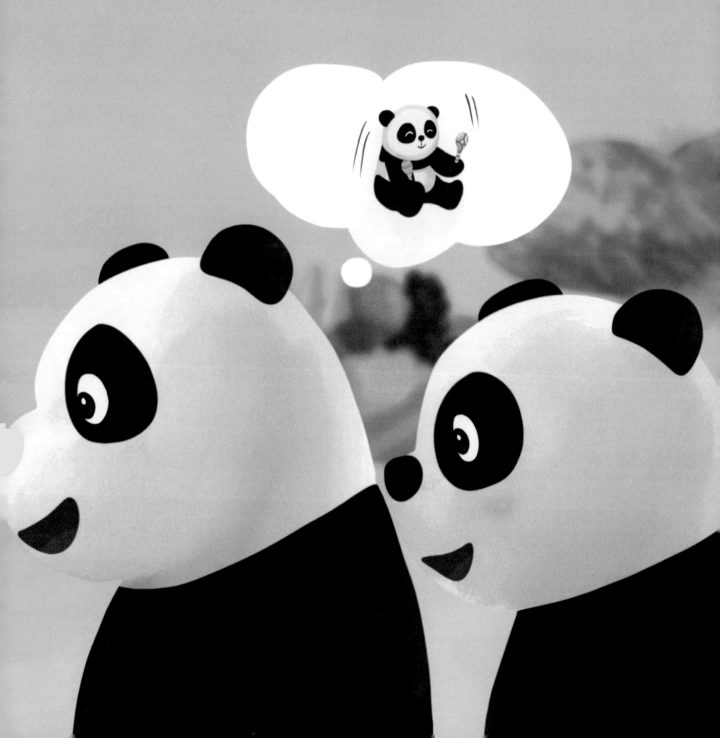

"I am glad you came to see me
Let's see what we can do.
I help animals grow their families.
I've helped pandas - just like you!"

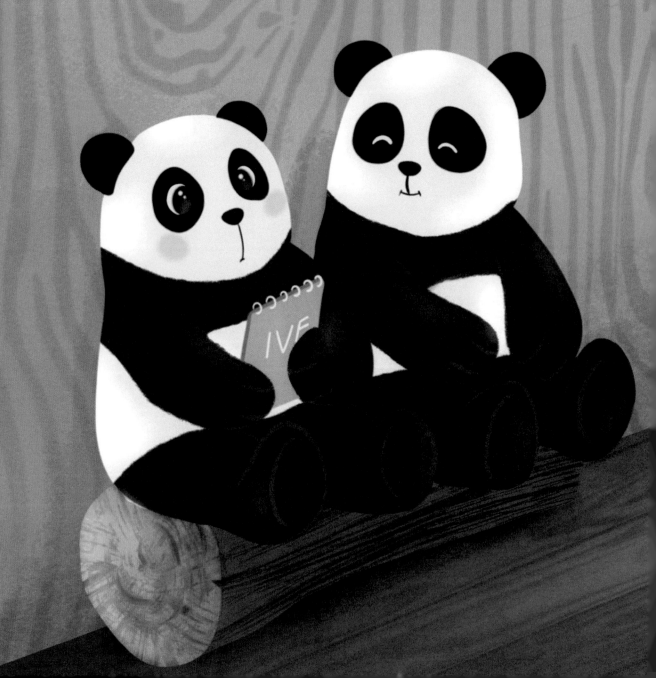

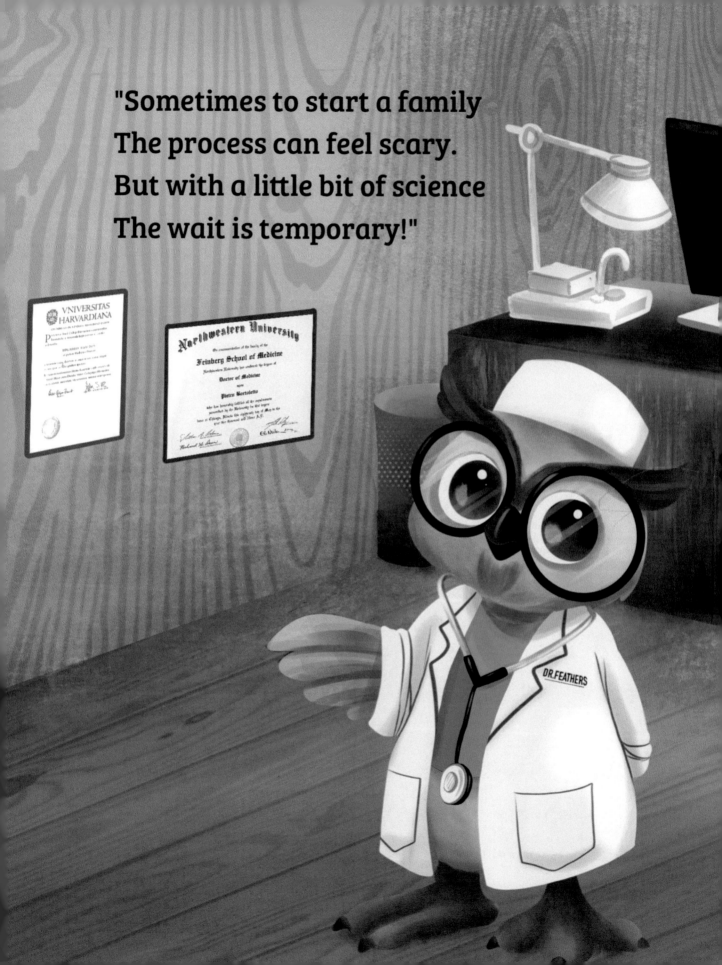

"Sometimes to start a family
The process can feel scary.
But with a little bit of science
The wait is temporary!"

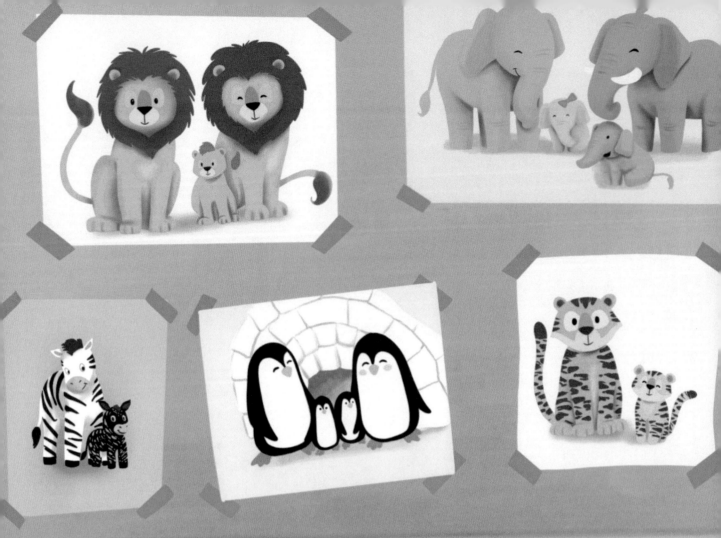

"All families are different.
They are made in different ways.
Some grow very easily,
And for others it feels like a maze."

Deb and Sue feel overwhelmed
They are just at the beginning.
The process ahead is daunting
But the outcome has them grinning!

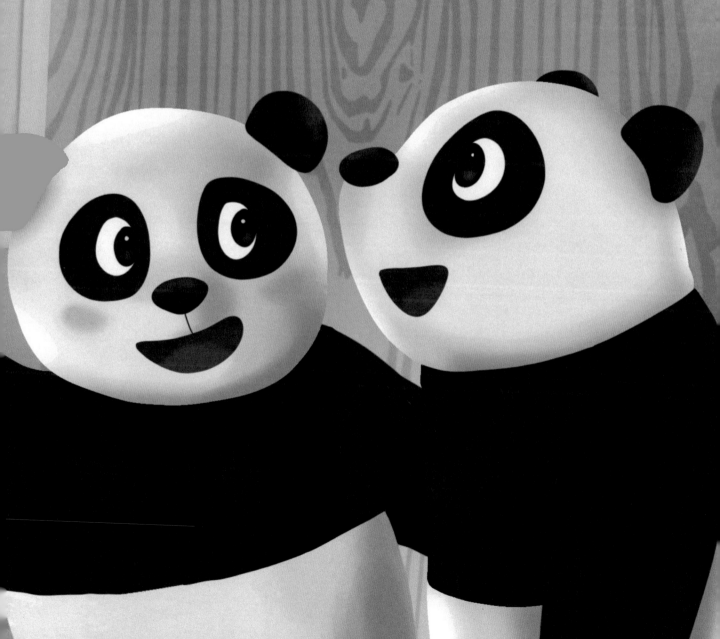

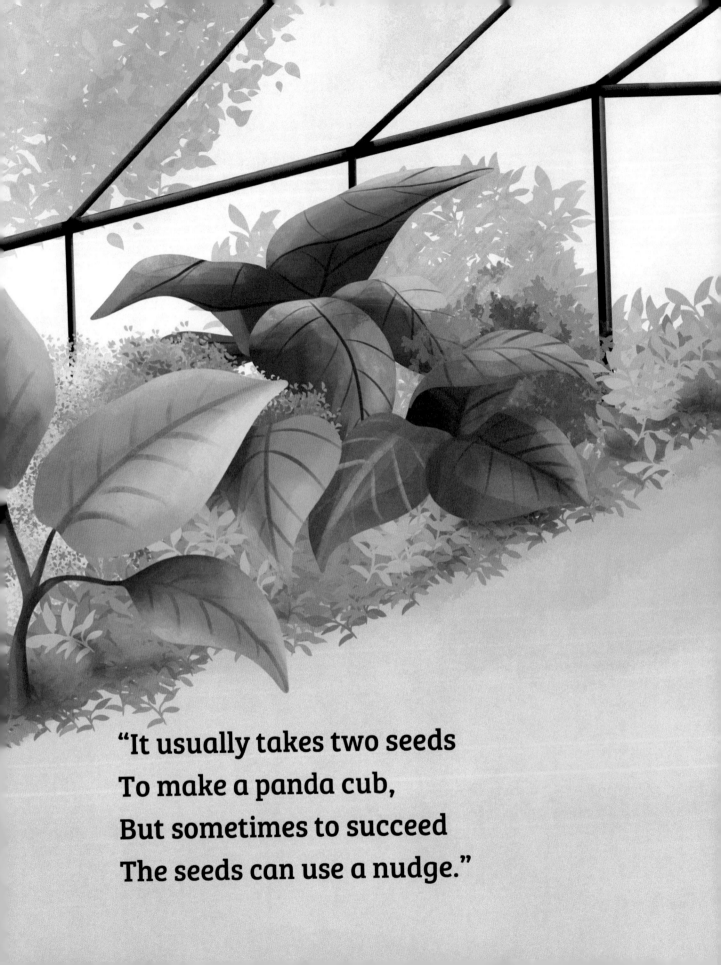

"It usually takes two seeds
To make a panda cub,
But sometimes to succeed
The seeds can use a nudge."

"When the time is right,
I'll plant them by each other.
With a bit of luck and lots of love
They will help make you both parents."

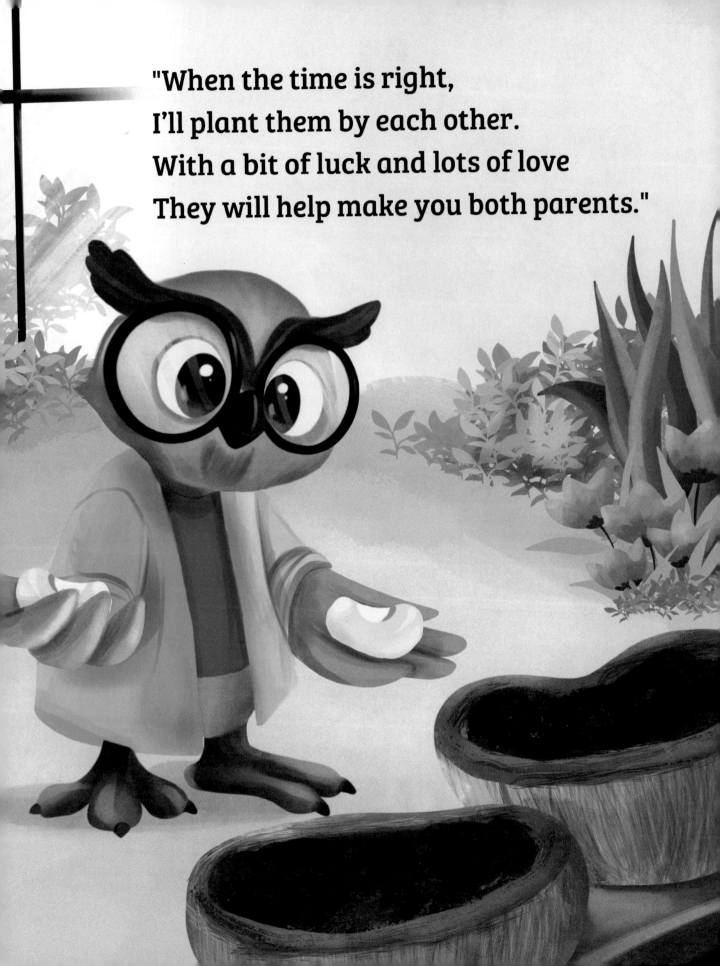

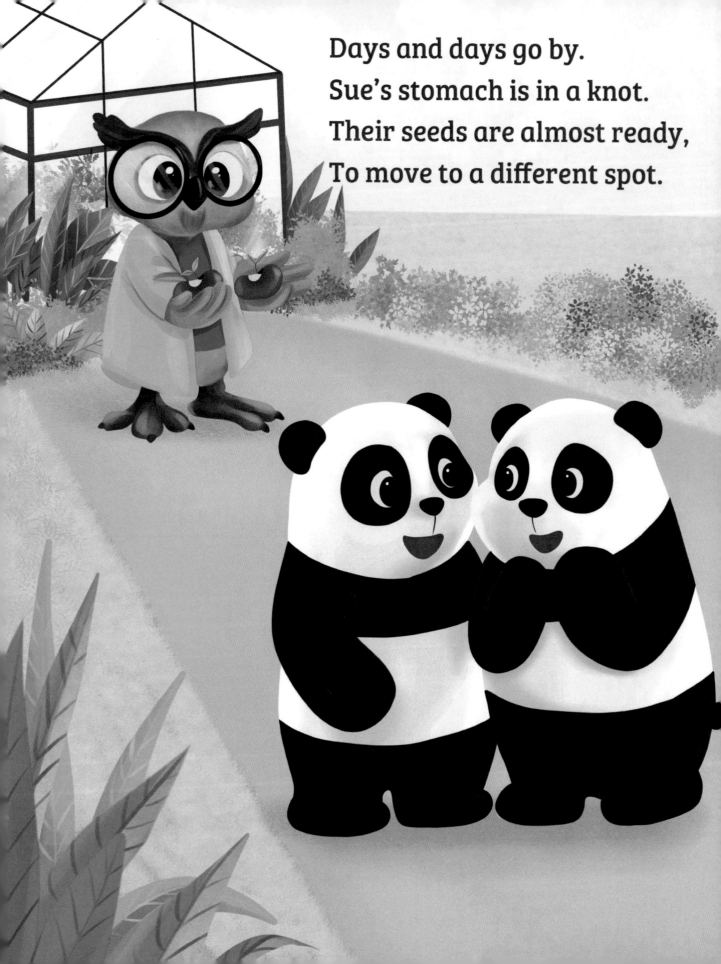

Days and days go by.
Sue's stomach is in a knot.
Their seeds are almost ready,
To move to a different spot.

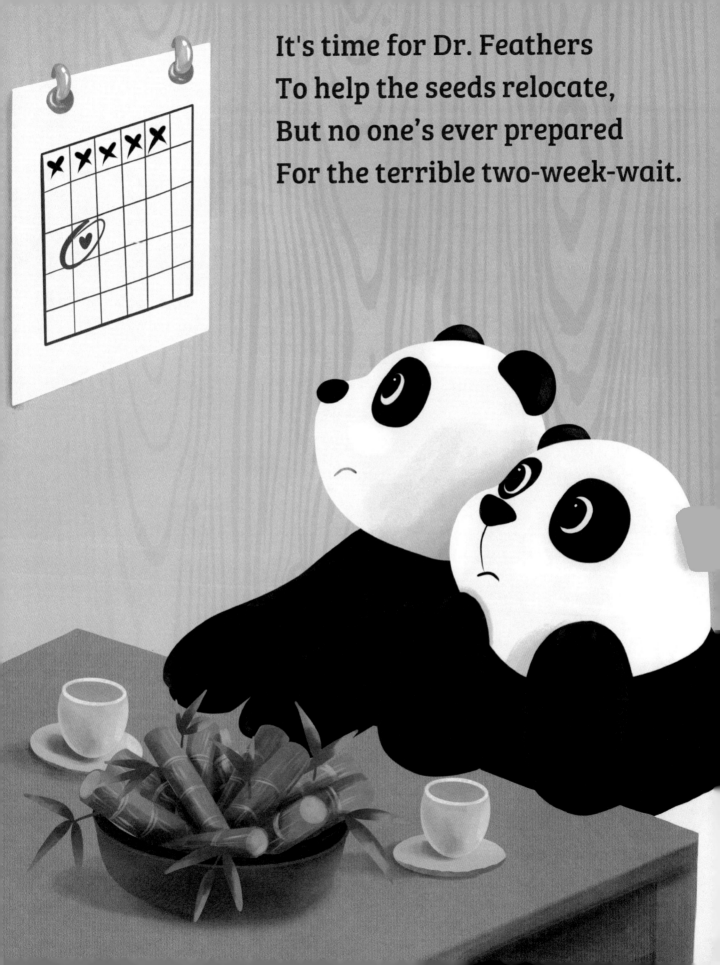

It's time for Dr. Feathers
To help the seeds relocate,
But no one's ever prepared
For the terrible two-week-wait.

It's time to check.
Could it really be?
Deb and Sue were once two
And now they will be three!

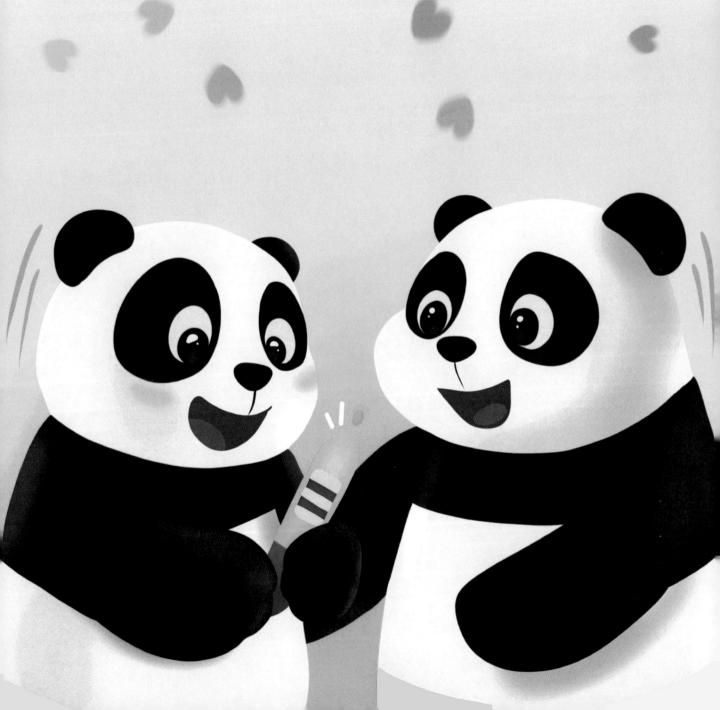

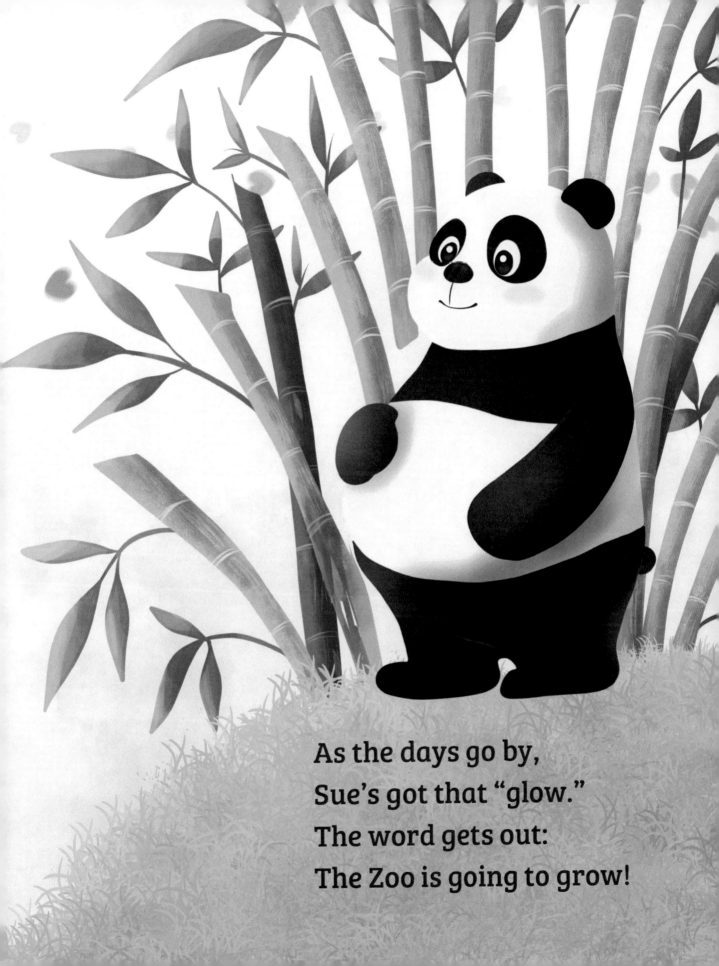

As the days go by,
Sue's got that "glow."
The word gets out:
The Zoo is going to grow!

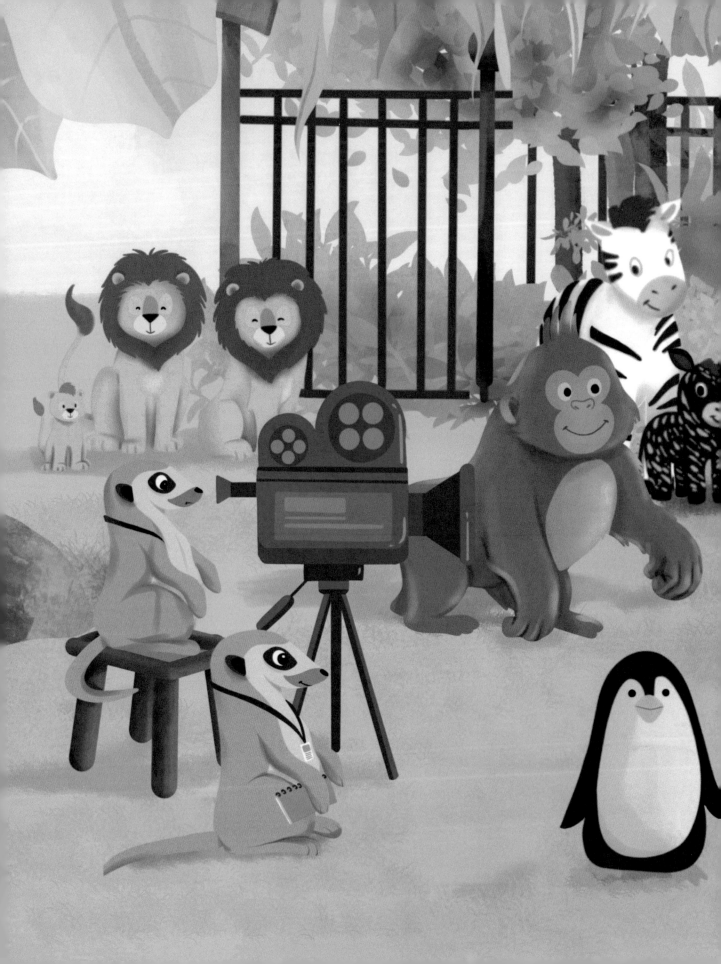

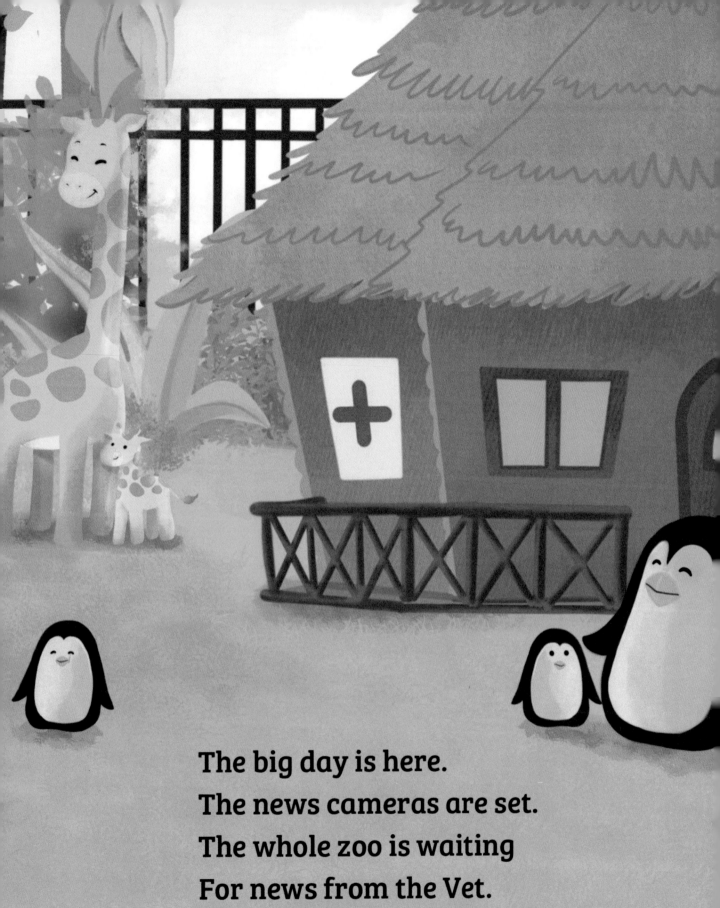

The big day is here.
The news cameras are set.
The whole zoo is waiting
For news from the Vet.

To their surprise,
It's two, not one!
Their once quiet life
Is about to get more fun.

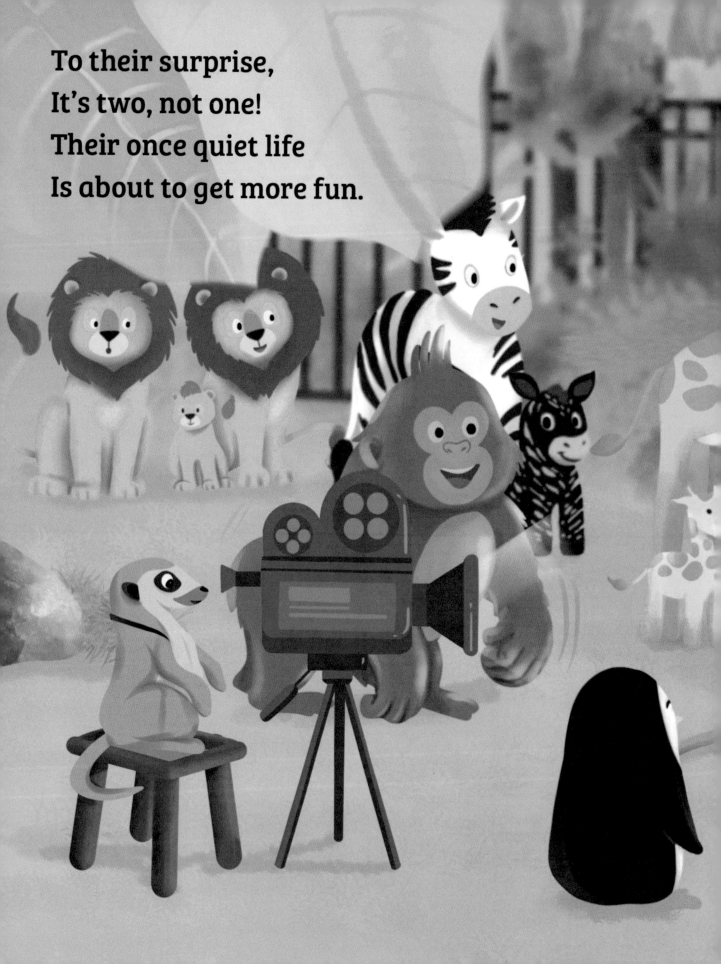

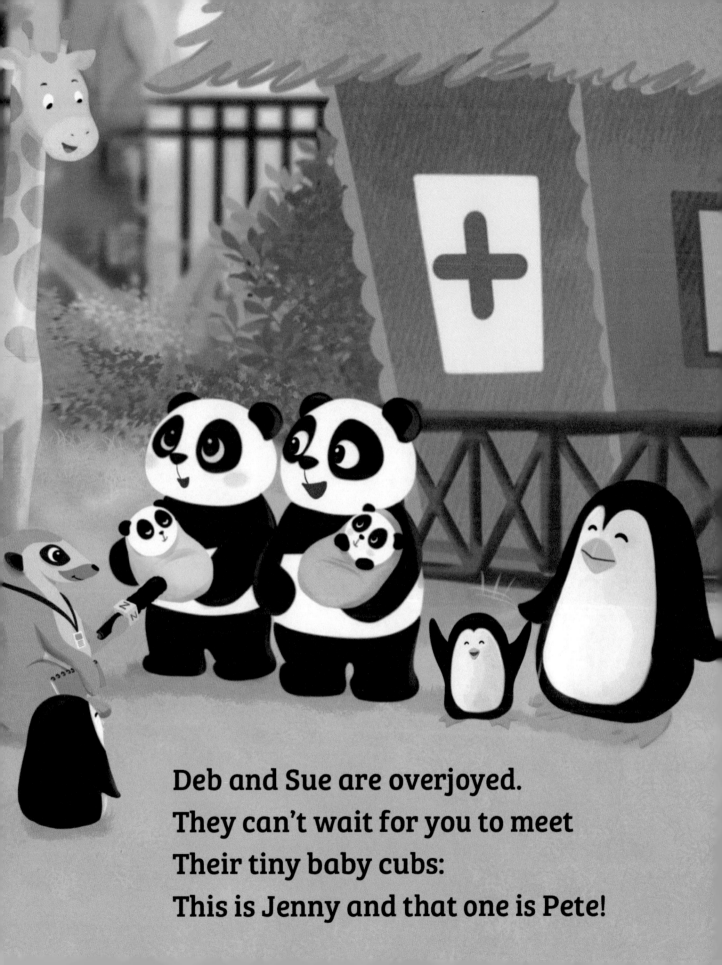

Deb and Sue are overjoyed.
They can't wait for you to meet
Their tiny baby cubs:
This is Jenny and that one is Pete!

Once upon a time
In the local city zoo
Lived a panda couple,
Whose dreams for a cub came true!

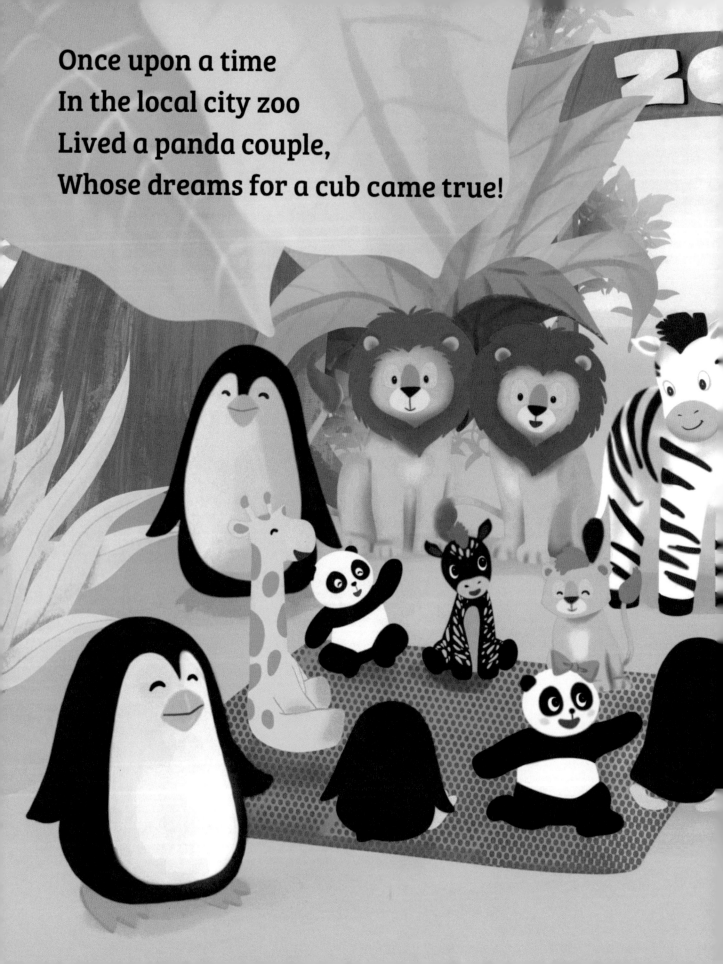

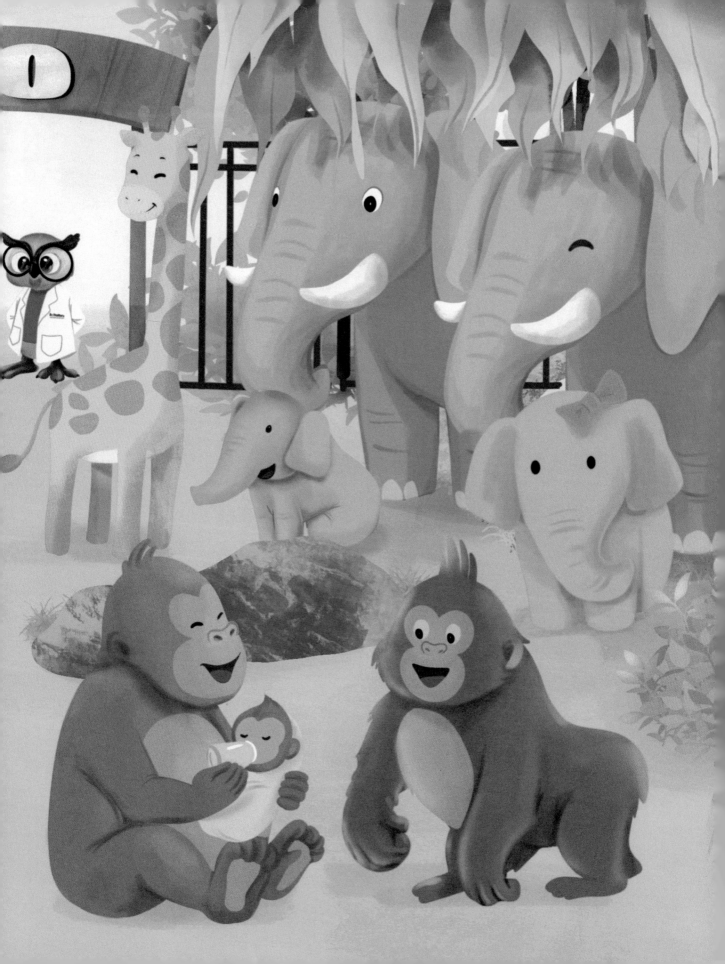

The End

Made in the USA
Middletown, DE
23 August 2024